Being Still in the Midst of Cancer

Being Still in the Midst of Cancer

✦

A Story of Faith, Friendship and Miracles

Rose Kronsperger
With Joan McPherson

iUniverse, Inc.
New York Lincoln Shanghai

Being Still in the Midst of Cancer
A Story of Faith, Friendship and Miracles

iUniverse, Inc.

For information address:
iUniverse, Inc.
2021 Pine Lake Road, Suite 100
Lincoln, NE 68512
www.iuniverse.com

ISBN: 0-595-31252-7

Printed in the United States of America

Contents

PREFACE

My name is Joan McPherson and on April 11, 2000 God reached down and touched my life. As a result, I will never be the same. His hand was in every aspect of the developing circumstances even though I sometimes had difficulty seeing it as I went through the ordeal that followed. Had it not been for His divine intervention, I don't believe I would be here today to tell my story.

Rose Kronsperger, who is my best friend and was my caregiver, has been kind enough to put my story to paper—writing it from my point of view.

While reading her Bible one day soon after my initial diagnosis, she came across Psalm 118: 17-18: "I will not die but live, and will proclaim what the Lord had done. The Lord has chastened me severely, but He has not given me over to death." These words would see us through some dark and difficult times and we would eventually see the power of the truth in them.

Throughout this experience we both kept journals and we have included excerpts from these at the beginning of each chapter. Several years ago we had decided to memorize a scripture verse each week. At the time we had no idea how much those verses would help us. Even though I had not been faithful in reviewing them, an appropriate one would come to mind at just the right time. Some of those verses appear throughout the book.

If you or someone you know is going through a similar experience, I pray this book will encourage you. Likewise, I pray that it will give you hope and inspire you to trust God no matter what happens—no matter what the circumstances may look like—because He has His eye on each of us and is intimately aware of and involved in everything that happens to us.

Technical note to the reader: Blood cells are produced in the bone marrow, the spongy tissue filling the center core of your bones. Each type of blood cell plays an important role in your body's normal function. These are the three types of blood cells:

1. Red blood cells carry oxygen to the tissues of the body. When your red blood cell count is low, your body tissues do not get enough oxygen to do their work. This results in a condition called anemia. The blood count test that measures anemia is called hemoglobin and/or hemat-

ocrit. For women, normal hemoglobin values are 11-15 g/dl and normal hematocrit values are 37-47

2. Platelets aid in the clotting of blood so that excessive bleeding is prevented when you hurt yourself. If there aren't enough platelets in your blood, you may bleed or bruise more easily than usual. Normal values are 140,000-450,000

3. White blood cells help to protect your body by fighting bacteria that cause infection. It is especially important to protect yourself against infection when your white blood cell count is low. Normal values are 3,500-10,000

1

"I know the plans I have for you," declares the Lord, "plans to prosper you and not to harm you, plans to give you hope and a future."
Jeremiah 29:11

THE DISCOVERY

I had been experiencing back pain for several weeks and thought it was nothing more than "getting older." I love to go for long walks but found that, because of the pain and discomfort, I could walk for only about 15 minutes before having to return home. I also had difficulty sleeping. I tried massage therapy (which only seemed to make matters worse) and eventually made an appointment with my doctor. He suggested some exercises, gave me a prescription for a muscle relaxant, and told me if it didn't improve in ten days he'd schedule me for physical therapy. Before that time passed, God began to move.

On a dark, rainy morning as I turned my car into the parking lot at work, I was hit by an oncoming car. The accident was not serious but because I was experiencing neck and chest pain and having difficulty breathing, the paramedics put a cervical collar on me and transported me to the hospital. Almost eight hours later tests and x-rays showed no apparent injuries. However, as I was preparing to leave I felt an excruciating pain in my stomach. Thinking it was from the seat belt (and because I just wanted to go home) I decided not to mention it to the doctor. But, again, God moved and the doctor entered the room just as I doubled over. He ordered a CT scan and an abnormal mass was found in my abdominal area. I tried to convince them (and myself) that it was probably scar tissue from gall bladder surgery I'd had 30 years ago, but they weren't convinced (primarily because it was on the wrong side) and scheduled a biopsy.

THE DIAGNOSIS

On Monday, April 24—the day after Easter—my primary physician called me at work and confirmed my worst fear: cancer! I was numb. I couldn't believe it! I went home and cried and prayed and cried some more. I had always said if I ever got cancer I didn't want to go through chemotherapy. In a hypothetical situation it had been easy to say what I would do—but now that the reality of it was staring me in the face, I wasn't so sure. I told Rose and we cried together. Then we talked and prayed about it and decided to at least explore my options.

I was fortunate to be working at a large pharmaceutical company at the time and had access to on-staff oncologists and researchers. They were invaluable in providing information and giving me a list of questions to ask the doctor. Once again, I realized that God had His hand in this and that it was no coincidence that I was working there at this particular time. I scheduled an appointment with an oncologist for that Friday. It was the first of many long weeks to come.

The doctor appointment is a blur to me now. Rose accompanied me with information she'd gotten on the Internet and the notes I had taken when talking to my co-workers. I heard the doctor speaking but didn't comprehend much of what he said. I just sat and stared at him with that "deer caught in the headlights" look. He advised us that it was serious but told us to be hopeful. As he spoke, Rose wrote furiously trying to get everything he said. I was glad she was there because I knew I wouldn't retain a word. I was completely overwhelmed.

I'd like to make a suggestion to anyone who has just been diagnosed with cancer or any serious illness. If possible, take someone with you when you go to your doctor appointments—preferably a close relative or good friend. Someone who can take notes, ask questions and keep a clear head because much of what is said will be difficult for you to recall later.

I was originally diagnosed with follicular center cell lymphoma. The tumor was approximately 7 centimeters long and 4 centimeters deep and was located in front of my left kidney near the abdominal aorta. It was blocking the left ureter from the kidney to the bladder and had, apparently, caused the kidney to shut down. Fortunately, God had allowed the cancer to be found early—my doctor told me it looked like it had only been there for about two months. I asked him if there was any way I could have anticipated or prevented this and he told me it was pretty much "the luck of the draw."

Initially, the diagnosis indicated that the cancer was probably low grade with different treatment options available including fairly mild intravenous chemotherapy over a 6-8 month period or possibly treatment in pill form for a year. The cancer would be a chronic condition and most likely never be completely gone but, hopefully, would go into remission. A bone marrow biopsy was scheduled for the following Friday, May 5, and a chest x-ray and CT scan the Tuesday after that. The biopsy had me quite nervous but I tried to rely on one of our learned verses: "God did not give us a spirit of fear, but of power, love and a sound mind" (2 Timothy 1:7). I was told that this type of lymphoma would almost certainly show up in the bone marrow. Even so, Rose and I prayed for the marrow to come back clear. Although I knew God was in control, I was anxious and, in the days that followed, tried in vain to immerse myself in my job.

The biopsy went well and when I got home from work on Wednesday, May 10 I rejoiced at the message on my answering machine: the marrow had come back clear—no evidence of lymphoma. I listened to it three times and fell to my knees praising and thanking Jesus—a direct answer to our prayers! My doctor ordered another core biopsy of the tumor to ascertain the grade and stage of the cancer.

At my next appointment on Wednesday, May 17 I learned that there was a change in the diagnosis. Even though the complete biopsy results were not yet in, the early findings showed that I had either an intermediate or high grade, large cell cancer. Although this diagnosis sounded worse than the original, it was actually better news. This cancer could be cured. The down side was that the chemotherapy would be intensive: 6-8 doses of something called "CHOP" chemo. There was an 80% chance that the tumor would be completely destroyed and if there was going to be a recurrence of the disease, it would be within the first two years.

It appeared that I would be able to receive my chemotherapy treatments at the outpatient clinic and, although I had hoped to continue working, I would have to take a medical leave of at least three months. Since I've always had bad reactions to prescription drugs, I was concerned about my reaction to the chemotherapy. My doctor did his best to reassure me that the anti-nausea drugs developed in recent years would provide some relief from the sickness-inducing poisons that were going to be pumped into me. My head was spinning as Rose and I left his office.

A LIFE TURNED UPSIDE DOWN

My first round of chemotherapy was scheduled for Friday, May 19 at 1:30 p.m. That morning, as I was preparing to leave for the clinic, the phone rang—it was my oncologist. He'd just received the rest of the biopsy results and the diagnosis had changed once again. He told me that I had a rare and aggressive type of non-Hodgkin's lymphoma: high grade, diffuse small noncleavel cell, called "Birkitt's" (less than 2% of all lymphomas are of this type.)

That changed everything. Instead of going to the clinic, he wanted me admitted to the hospital. The treatment protocol also changed drastically. I would be receiving massive amounts of chemotherapy—including Cytoxan, Cytosar, Adriamycin and Methotrexate—in six rounds of treatment, each one requiring a hospital stay of 5-7 days. I would also have to endure several intrathecal injections—spinal taps with injections of chemotherapy drugs directly into the spine. My doctor informed me that this type of cancer sometimes works its way into the spinal fluid and then into the brain. Ironically, he had recently treated another patient with this same diagnosis. In my heart I knew it was no coincidence that he was my doctor.

At the end of the day on Friday, May 19—less than one month after the initial diagnosis—I found myself in the hospital facing a very frightening future. In five weeks' time my entire life had been turned upside down and I had no guarantee that I was going to come out of it alive.

As I reflect on the early weeks after discovering I had cancer and enduring all those tests, I believe God gave me a very calm spirit to deal with everything I faced. It wasn't an absence of fear or concern, but I believe this is where I experienced the "peace that passes all understanding" (Phil. 4:6-7). When I became anxious, I would recite verses and try to hear His still, small voice. Sometimes I would hear it, sometimes not. Going through the extensive testing was unnerving—not only because of the actual procedures, but also because the waiting was so difficult. And, of course, my verse for those times was the verse that's been with me since I became a Christian: "Be still and know that I am God." I also recited Psalm 91 many times, especially during the first biopsy and the subsequent core and bone marrow biopsies. I saw God's fingerprints all over these things.

2

"And we know that God causes everything to work together for the good of those who love God and are called according to His purpose for them."
Romans 8:28 (New Living Translation)

Journal Entry—Sunday, May 21, 2000[1]

This is my first week in the hospital. I had anticipated my first treatment to be yesterday—NOT! Apparently with this sort of chemotherapy protocol, which is extremely intense, my body needs a little "prepping" which happened yesterday. First treatment was today so I got up early and spent some time reading my Bible. The treatment went very well which is fairly surprising to me since I react pretty negatively to drugs of any sort and have been concerned about the chemo stories I've heard. I didn't even get sick.

Tuesday, May 23

What a difference a day makes! Yesterday was the total opposite of Sunday. I was pretty sick. I had to have my second spinal tap and my doctor had a difficult time finding spinal fluid. Needless to say, this is not a pleasant experience any time it's done but it was especially painful because he had to try two different places and still couldn't tap in successfully. I had been praying that it would go as well as the one on Friday, but no such luck. He didn't want to cause me any more pain so he said he'd try again today (oh, yay! Something to look forward to!) I also had a port put in for my treatments. (A port is a device they insert under the skin to take the chemo directly so they don't have to keep searching for veins since chemotherapy does a job on your veins too!)

I've been quite nervous but the spinal tap today went pretty well. The fluid is still clear—thank you, Jesus! I was glad to get that over with. Satan's been in my face but I tried to remember, "The Lord is close to the broken hearted and saves those who are crushed in spirit" (Psalm 34:18). I've been feeling pretty sick again today and know that the "fall out" of my hair will start soon. I dread it with all my heart but Rose has arranged for me to pick out a couple of wigs and hats so I'll have them when it does happen. I think I may get to go home tomorrow. I sure hope so especially since I know I have to come back in on Sunday for the next round!

---

1. All journal entries are from my journal except where noted.

MY NEW ORBIT

The Oncology wing of the hospital was like a little universe of its own. There was a small kitchen with a refrigerator where I could have my own food brought in, labeled and stored. The freezer was supplied with ice cream and popsicles. Adjacent to the kitchen was a lounge with a small library, a TV, some videos and an automated reclining chair that I particularly liked. Beyond the nurse's station, through the double doors and down a short hall was the chapel, where I often went when I needed solitude and quiet. Although the busy activities of the hospital were going on right around the corner, it seemed a million miles away. A small courtyard outside the chapel was a comforting place to pray and listen to the birds.

There was another courtyard right outside the Oncology unit. Sometimes as I was sitting there, one of the other cancer patients would come out and light up a cigarette. I find it difficult to comprehend how someone who is fighting this horrible disease can continue to smoke. Although I certainly understand the difficulty in breaking a habit (I've struggled with more than a few), to be in the midst of chemotherapy and yet continue to indulge in something so deadly baffles me.

I'm not sure which was worse: not knowing what was coming or knowing and anticipating it. My first stay in the hospital was unnerving since I really didn't know what to expect. Each day brought a new occasion for concern and trepidation. But overall, the first round of treatment and the five-day hospital stay went pretty well. During future treatments I became accustomed to the routine and procedures but it didn't alleviate the anxiety. Facing the unknown is always frightening—and sometimes we also fear what we know is coming.

Rose became my caregiver and made the commitment to stay with me through the entire process. Once home, we quickly developed a routine that would continue throughout the next four months. I needed to take so many drugs that she decided to keep a notebook citing each drug, the dosage and the time it was taken in order to keep it all straight. Day after day the litany was repeated: Diflucan, Darvocet, Flexeril, Lorazepam, Cipro, Allopurinal, Zofran. By the end of this ordeal we had completely filled a 3" x 5" memo book. Knowing my history of reactions to prescription drugs, I prayed for God's protection. Even though Rose and I were very scared, we continued to hang onto Jesus and the truth and promise of His word. The tests of trust and faith were just beginning and we prayed that rather than fall into the temptation to despair, we would stay strong and steadfast. This was certainly the most difficult thing either of us had ever had to face.

Since coming to faith in Christ in 1976 we each had, of course, endured our share of tests and hardships. The hard reality of death had visited me early in my walk with Jesus: one of my brothers had died unexpectedly just six months after I had become a Christian and then Rose's father and mine died within two years of each other. Another two years after that my family learned that my mother had cancer. This began a five-year struggle that resulted in her death in 1989. Eleven years later I was facing this deadly disease and my own mortality.

FACING A SCARY FUTURE

When the daylight of good health becomes the long, dark night of illness, time seems to stand still. The reality of the situation hits and you know you have to deal with it but your thought process doesn't work very well. Even the smallest decisions are difficult and you find yourself stumbling through the days, going through the motions but not really conscious of what you're doing. Each day you do what's required and then lie awake through the long night trying not to think about what's happening to you, what may be coming and how you'll get through it. Sleep can either be as elusive as trying to capture the wind or it can be a wonderful escape, but there was no escaping this situation. Often I couldn't sleep and even when I did it invaded my dreams.

A blessing is often preceded by a period of testing. The brightest morning must sometimes be preceded by the darkest night. I had to learn this and it was to be a difficult lesson—one that would test the very limits of my faith and endurance. God was going to kick out all the props I was leaning on so that all I could do was lean on Him. This is, I think, one of the most valuable lessons a Christian can learn and one that is only learned through adversity. God does not want us to be strong and independent. He doesn't help those who help themselves. He helps the weak and needy—those of us who admit that we mess things up and that a particular situation is way beyond our abilities. When we do this and call on Him for help, we can experience the all-sufficient grace of God and the strength only He can give. We can know the "peace that passes all understanding" and the comforting assurance that the Ancient of Days is working in every detail on our behalf. This doesn't take away the anxiety or the fear—we're human beings and these feelings are normal. But the knowledge that God is in control allows us to go beyond what we feel and move into the area of trust. It's a narrow, rocky road but as long as we remember that He's right beside us, it's a road we know we can walk.

3

"Be still and know that I am God."
Psalm 46:10

Journal Entry—Wednesday, May 24, 2000

I'm home and so happy to be here! I fell to my knees and thanked Jesus through a few tears while Rose was bringing my stuff in from the car. I just don't know how I would get through this without her. She has been a rock for me to lean on. I just hope I don't lean too hard on her and not enough on Jesus.

Being home is wonderful. I've actually been able to eat a little fried rice and some macaroni and cheese and keep it down. The chemo is starting to affect my taste buds. I slept a lot today and being in my own bed was heavenly!

Thursday, May 25

Today we picked out a couple of wigs and I got my hair cut short—trying to prepare myself for what's coming. The wigs are a good match and very close to the color and style of my hair. I was pretty wiped out by the time we got home and feeling a little sick. It's great being home even if all I can do is sit in my chair and look out the window.

HOME SWEET HOME

The time spent at home between my treatments was a refuge. Even though I was weak and couldn't do much more than sit in my recliner chair watching TV, listening to music or just looking out the window, it was a joy to be out of the hospital and have even a <u>little</u> sense of normalcy! I took frequent naps while Rose was at work. My daily routine was quite basic: get up, read my Bible, sit in the living room and doze while watching TV. Lunch usually consisted of oatmeal and toast and then I'd lie down for a while and take a nap. I always felt a little better when Rose got home from work. It was unnerving being home alone with too much time to think—and managing all the pills I had to take was confusing and tiring. Rose did a good job of keeping me on track and, at times, was like a drill sergeant, scolding me when I tried to do too much.

One of the many difficult things about my hospital stays was the bed. Even though I had my own pillow (which was a great help), I had a lot of trouble getting comfortable and rarely got a good night's sleep. Rose tried to solve the problem by showing up one day carrying a foam mattress pad. It seemed to make things a little more tolerable and I appreciated her thoughtfulness. I'm sure it was quite comical to see us coming into the hospital each time I was admitted carrying this rolled up mass of pink foam for my bed!

I was beginning to lose my taste for food but it was nothing compared to what was to come. I did my best to enjoy what I could. Tea and toast, oatmeal, fried rice and macaroni and cheese seemed to be the most appealing at this stage. Later, I wouldn't be able to tolerate even that.

I found myself doing some self-examination regarding my imminent hair loss. I wondered if perhaps God was dealing with my vanity and pride. I had always been a little obsessed with how my hair looked and had spent a lot of time and money on perms, highlights and styling. Later, when I had completely lost my hair, I'd look in the mirror and hardly recognize myself. I guess I was finally learning that looks don't define a person—it's what's on the inside. I was still the same person in my heart whether or not I had hair.

TOO MUCH OF A GOOD THING

I tried to go outside whenever possible—especially when I was in the hospital, even if it meant dragging my IV pole along with me. I took advantage of the courtyard outside the Oncology wing as often as I could. I didn't have to walk too far, and could still be outside. Enjoying the flowers and birds was a nice diversion and helped pass the time. I had to be careful, however, as the chemotherapy drugs make you extremely sensitive to the sun. I learned that lesson one particularly nice day when I spent a little too much time outside. I decided to go for a walk and, since I went a little further than I should have, was out for a fairly long time. When I got back to my room my nurse came in, peered at me over the top of her glasses with a reprimanding look and told me that I needed to be very careful of sun exposure. I looked in the mirror and saw why she was upset: my cheeks were much rosier than they should have been—as was the whole side of my face! When my doctor came in later that day, he laughed and said, "I see you got a little color." When I told him I had already been chastised, he also warned me about sun exposure and advised me to wear a wide-brimmed hat if I was going to be outside for any length of time.

Walking has always been a favorite pastime of mine and I was determined not to let this ordeal rob me of that. I went for short walks when at home and even walked around the hospital grounds. There, however, I always had my trusty IV pole—but I didn't let that stop me! My walks started out tentative and short both in duration and distance, but as I became more and more confident (and homesick) they got longer and further. Each day I covered a little more distance than the day before. It got to the point where I was walking out to one of the roads leading into the hospital. Rose once told my nurse that I was inching my way home and one of these days would make a break and run for it! We laughed at the picture of me in my pajamas skulking furtively down the road as I made my escape, dragging an IV pole and trying to look inconspicuous!

GOOD FRIENDS

Rose and I both believed in God's faithfulness even though it was hard to see as we looked down the long, hard road before us. Every day we endeavored to try to see only the path we walked that day and not the entire journey. What appeared to be bad now could turn out good. I thought of the story in the Old Testament about Joseph and his comment to his brothers: "What you meant for my harm, God has made for my good." He certainly wasn't able to see that very clearly (if at all) while he was a slave and in prison. Only after he was raised to his position of authority, did he see the purpose of what he had experienced. He grew in character and wisdom during his trials. I fervently prayed that I would not do less. I often thought of Romans 5:3-5 which says, "...but we also rejoice in our sufferings, because we know that suffering produces perseverance; perseverance, character; and character, hope. And hope does not disappoint us, because God has poured out his love into our hearts by the Holy Spirit, whom he has given us."

Having a close relative or good friend to help you during something like this is a wonderful gift—you need and want their help. I found that knowing our limitations and reaching out to others for support is not a sign of weakness but of strength. My immediate support came from my family and best friend. The support I received from other friends—in the form of cards, books, flowers and gifts—was very touching. I now have quite a collection of small, stuffed bears that were sent to me during this time. I also received "care packages" of tea, soup and pudding. Receiving a card with a short note of encouragement would brighten my day. Rose sent email updates almost daily to my friends at work, and during their lunch break some would visit me at the hospital or at home. There would come a time, however, when I would not want them to see me—not because I didn't want visitors, but because of the way I looked and felt.

I also received cards from people I barely knew, touched that someone who didn't even know me very well would send a card or write a short note of encouragement. These are small things that all of us can do for others but we often just don't take the time. I've been guilty of that more times than I'd like admit; but I now realize how uplifting something so simple can be. Little acts of kindness become jewels in heavenly crowns.

4

"I will call on God, and the Lord will rescue me. Morning, noon, and night I plead aloud in my distress, and the Lord hears my voice. He rescues me and keeps me safe from the battle waged against me, even though many still oppose me."
Psalm 55:16-18 (NLT)

Journal Entry—Monday, May 29

The days I was home really flew by—nothing like they drag here in the hospital. I'm back for my second round of chemotherapy. It's still hard for me to believe this is happening, but just knowing that God is still in control comforts my heart.

Of course, I also see Satan and his armies trying to distract and discourage me. This morning I spilled some juice on the floor and realized this was just an attempt to stop me from doing my reading. So instead of giving in, I sent Jesus to handle it as I tried to keep a quiet attitude and moved my IV pole in and out of the bathroom getting paper towels to clean up the mess. It's now 7:30 a.m. and I already have a pretty good headache. Not a great way to start the day. My meds and breakfast should be coming soon.

This is the 24-hour treatment and I'm pretty nervous about it. I checked into the hospital around 7:00 p.m. yesterday so they could hydrate me for 12 hours before starting the chemo attack. This time it's high doses of methotrexate for 21 hours followed by what they call a Lukavoran rescue where they flush out all the chemo and wait for the toxicity levels to drop back down. This isn't a fun time and already I can't wait to go home.

Wednesday, May 31

I received two blood transfusions today and was quite scared. My nurse and I said a prayer over the blood and I recited Exodus 14:13-14: "Do not be afraid; stand firm and you will see the deliverance the Lord will bring you today. The Lord will fight for you; you need only to be still." Even though I appeared calm, I was shaking inside and tried to recall more verses. One I remembered was, "Lord, when doubts fill my mind and my heart is in turmoil, quiet me, and give me renewed hope and cheer." (Psalm 94:19)

Rose left work early today ("on a hunch") and came up to spend the day. I'm so glad she did! This hasn't been a very good day. The nurses here are great, though. I've had a bit of an attitude because I want to go home and was told "maybe tomorrow."

Thursday morning, June 1

So far, this has been a bad day all around—took a shower and my hair is really falling out. I knew this would be hard, but I'm sure it would help if only I could be at home. My blood work is the determining factor on that and it's not due in until around 3:00 p.m. I'm trusting Jesus to let me go. My nurse seems to think I'm here for the night and is talking about my 3:30 meds! I keep asking her to call the doctor to find out.

Thursday evening

No sooner did Rose leave than the nurse came in and told me I could go home! Thank you, Jesus! I called Rose and asked her to come back and pick me up, even though it was around 7:00 p.m. I wanted out! What a surprise when I got home: there, in my living room, was a new couch! I love it and will be able to rest without going to bed all the time.

The blessing was coming home and the new couch. Then the trial came with the prescriptions they sent home with me. At the hospital pharmacy, Rose was told that the drugs prescribed weren't covered by my insurance and that one was going to cost $5,000 and the other $2,000. She came home empty-handed and frustrated. We're both tired and upset but realize there isn't anything we can do about it tonight anyhow, so we prayed and left it in God's hands. We reminded ourselves that He knew what was going on and all we had to do was trust Him to straighten it out. Sometimes we just can't seem to see God in any of this—and yet we know He's in it everywhere. So we just hang on, believe and trust Him to work it all out. We do what we can and let Him take care of the rest.

Friday, June 2

We checked with my doctor today and, after spending 3 hours at the pharmacy, finally got all the prescriptions for $34. (The mix-up was due to a computer glitch!) Thank you again, Jesus!

Monday, June 5

I've been home three days and it's been wonderful. Yesterday, though, I had to call my friend Sandy and ask her to cut what's left of my hair really short. It's mostly gone now and I'm beginning my "wig period." This is so difficult. I'll be glad when it's over. I'm finding that I'm grateful for even the smallest things, like being able to go for two 30-minute walks with Rose today—a slow pace but better than I've been able to do in months! It's just great to be able to be outside!

Friday, June 9

Saw my doctor today. I had blood work done on Monday, Wednesday and again today before my appointment with him. On Monday my white count was 80, on Wednesday it was up to 400 and today it was at 1,400. He's very pleased with this so he's putting me back in the hospital tomorrow for the next round. My reward. I guess, for bouncing back! At least I don't have to check in until around 9:00 p.m.

ROUND TWO

The nausea I felt with the second treatment was more like what I had anticipated and I found that I was even more scared. I desperately tried to hang on to the verses I had memorized. It was amazing how many of them applied to my current situation. I tried to remind myself that when I was learning them 4-5 years ago, God had already known I'd need them now. It gave me some comfort but it was still a very frightening time.

Rose had decided this whole situation called for new furniture. My living room was pretty small and was furnished with only a couple of reclining chairs and my mother's rocking chair. The chemotherapy was making me very tired and whenever I wanted to lie down, I had to go to bed. So she decided to get rid of the two chairs and buy a couch with recliners on each end. She arranged for it to be delivered while I was in the hospital. Things worked out perfectly—it was delivered the morning I was released. Again we saw God watching over our every-day activities and smoothing the road before us—even in the little things like a couch delivery!

HEALTH CONCERNS

Because of my low blood levels due to the chemotherapy, I had to start giving myself injections to increase my red and white blood cells. These were the pre-scriptions Rose had difficulty filling and were added to all the other drugs I was taking. I had to have a Neupogen injection every day and Epogen once a week. There was no way Rose could do this for me. She gets queasy around needles and would have been shaking so badly I didn't particularly trust her. I knew I had to do it myself. She was, however, able to at least prepare the syringe but as for the injection itself—it was up to me. It's surprising what you can do when you know you have to! If I had thought about it at any other time, I don't think I could have done it. But when it comes to something as serious as blood levels, I found that you get the strength to do what you have to in order to stay as healthy as pos-sible. God's strength was there in my weakness.

During the entire treatment process—which lasted about 4 months—my temperature was closely monitored. Because of the assault on the immune system by the chemotherapy, the risk of infections and other illnesses is high. When I was discharged that Thursday, the nurse told me that if my temperature went over 100 I was to call the doctor or get back to the hospital. While Rose was at the pharmacy trying to get my prescriptions filled I took my temperature—it was 101. I told myself that it was only spiking because of the activity and excitement of getting out of the hospital and I decided not to tell her when she got home. I'm surprised I got away with it—but I guess she was so frustrated about the prescriptions she didn't notice the guilty look on my face. We took my temperature later and it had gone down to 99. Once more, I thanked God for His mercy and care.

For the past 25 years I have made an effort to eat healthy and take vitamin supplements regularly. This, I think, was very helpful in my ability to bounce back from the chemotherapy treatments. Being in pretty good health—except for the tumor—was a definite advantage. I believe that these years of preparation were instrumental in my recovery. My blood levels rebounded well with the injections, and my doctor decided that I was ready for the third round. After that, he said I'd probably get about three weeks to recuperate and then we'd do it all over again. I didn't care for that part of it, but the three-week break sounded wonderful! I decided to hang onto that to help me get through the next hospital stay.

PERSONAL STRUGGLES

My hair loss was very upsetting, as I knew it would be. It's a traumatic experience. (I also lost my eyebrows and eyelashes.) When there wasn't much left, I asked my friend who's a hairdresser to cut it very short. At one point I was so upset I thought of having her shave my head and be done with it, but she convinced me to let her just cut it. Even so, when I got home I wished I'd gone ahead and had it shaved. The actual process of losing my hair was, I think, worse than having it completely gone. I supposed my reasoning was, once it's gone, it's gone—at least I won't have to have it coming out every time I wash it. Anyone who's gone through this knows what I'm talking about. Taking clumps of hair from your pillow in the morning is no way to start your day.

I'd heard that many people who lost their hair through chemotherapy had it grow back a totally different texture—even a different color. I hoped for curly hair since mine had been stick straight all my life. I didn't care much about what color it might be. As I went through the months with my head as bald as a billiard ball, I anticipated the day I'd see it start to grow and looked forward to having a full head of hair again. Everyone assured me that it would come back—and I knew it would—but when I looked in the mirror each morning it was hard to believe. I remembered reading that God had the very hairs on our head numbered and I had to laugh when I thought about my current count!

When I was home, the ability to go for a walk—especially without dragging an IV pole with me—was a real treat. I found myself treasuring small things like this that I had taken for granted just a few months before. Although I felt that I was missing the entire spring and summer, I was also grateful that this was happening when the weather was nice and I was able to be outside for short periods of time even when I was in the hospital. Instead of looking at the down side of things, I made a decision to look at the positive things I was able to do. This helped immensely and provided an opportunity to slow down and become more aware of the little things we usually miss in our busy daily lives.

5

*"Let the morning bring me word of your unfailing love, for I have put my trust in you.
Show me the way I should go, for to you I lift up my soul."*
Psalm 143:8

<u>*Journal Entry—Sunday, June 11*</u>

*Here I am back in for another chemo onslaught today through Wednesday with, hope-
fully, release on Thursday. Please, Lord, keep my blood counts good so I can go home
on Thursday.*

*So far, Sunday has been pretty uneventful. I started feeling a little nauseous while
getting the chemo but they gave me some Compazine and I slept for a couple of hours.
My sleeping patterns here are weird. I don't sleep that well at night since they wake me
up every couple of hours to take vitals and check on me. So I end up taking catnaps
during the day and getting my rest when I can. I felt bad sending Rose home today
because I was so tired but I know she understands.*

*I see a man sitting in the courtyard and took the opportunity to pray for him. God
knows his story (I don't need to) and I know prayers always help. Nancy, one of my
nurses who had breast cancer, was on duty today and we had a chance to talk about
the Lord. It really helps to talk to someone who has been through a similar experience.
She told me that after her chemo was over she missed the grace and love she felt from
God during that time and had started to depend on herself again. I understood what
she meant. After my head injury seven years ago, I counted on Jesus so much for each
day and when I went back to work I really missed the quiet time I had established
with Him. I hope that when this is over I continue to make a quiet time with Jesus.*

*Rose told me that she and our friend Derl are binding my arms to theirs and
they're taking the roles of Aaron and Hur (see Exodus 17). They're claiming the victory over the enemy: Jesus over the cancer as Joshua defeated the Amalekites. I have so
many people praying for me. Sometimes I think I can actually <u>feel</u> the power of their
prayers.*

<u>*Monday, June 12*</u>

*I had a pretty good night's sleep last night but woke up this morning with a terrible
headache. I'm scheduled for an ultrasound some time today for my kidney. I pray
everything is all right.*

Well, no sooner did I write that than they came to take me for an ultrasound of my pancreas, abdominal aorta and both kidneys. The doctor will be in later today to go over the results. I read this morning in Psalms: "Who have I in heaven but you; and earth has nothing I desire besides you"—so, Father in heaven, please give me a good report.

Tuesday, June 13

Not a good day today: got sick first thing this morning—not the way I wanted to start my day. I'm taking more anti-nausea meds and they seem to be helping. Karen and Pam came to see me today. That was nice—broke my day up a little. Mary [my sister] stopped in too, brought me a chocolate shake and we sat outside for a little while. Rose came later also, of course—she's here every day and I always look forward to seeing her. I'm hoping I can go home tomorrow but I'm not sure about that.

Wednesday, June 14

John [my brother] is coming to visit today. I'm looking forward to seeing him. I'm still waiting to have another spinal tap. It was scheduled for around 9:00 a.m. but it's already 10:40 and nothing yet. The anticipation is unsettling. I just pray that whenever it happens, it goes well. "The angel of the Lord camps around those who fear Him and He delivers them." (Psalm 34:7) I have an angel camped around me!
(later that same day)
   My spinal went real well (thank you, Jesus!) so that waiting is over. It was around 2:15 p.m. when they finally did it. My oncologist is on vacation so I had a different one do it this time. She used a smaller needle and the procedure seemed to go better. Whatever the reason, I'm glad that part is over no matter who does it!
   I've slept a lot today which is good but I'm not thinking too clearly. When they brought dinner at 6:00 p.m. I though it was morning and they were bringing me breakfast! All the drugs I'm on seem to be messing with my head a little.

Thursday, June 15

I feel pretty good this morning. It's only 9:30 but so far, today is really dragging—probably because I'm so anxious to go home! I'm still waiting to hear from the doctor. Her schedule sure is different than my regular doctor—he's usually in here around 6:30 a.m.! I feel better today than when I saw her yesterday. She thought I looked "a little punk"—probably just the turban!

It's now 11:00, my last chemo has been hung and I'm still waiting to see the doctor.

(later that same day)

Finally got the word: I'm out of here! Thank you, Jesus! I just want to go home, get out of these pajamas and sit on my new couch for a while! I get a three-week reprieve—a little time to get back on my feet before we start all over again.

ROUND THREE

This third time in the hospital was much more difficult. I didn't want to go back and that set the stage for impatient frustration. I was already tired of the whole ordeal and it was hard not to dread the three more rounds of chemo I faced. Since it would be a complete repeat of what I'd just been through, I pretty much knew what to expect—and I wasn't looking forward to going through it all over again! However, I tried not to look that far ahead but only toward the three-week break that lay before me. It looked almost as good as a vacation (though not quite) and I prayed I would continue to get stronger and that my blood levels would come back to a relatively normal count.

LESSONS AND DISTRACTIONS

During this time I reflected almost daily on what was happening to me and how I could grow from it. I only allowed myself to ask "why?" after the initial diagnosis. Realizing I might never know the answer, I decided not to dwell on the "why" but to focus my energy on getting through it and getting better. I relied daily on the strength of my faith. I remembered the words from a song by Rich Mullins: "when your faith gets shaken, sometimes your heart gets stirred." I had always liked that line but this experience gave me a real understanding of the truth of it. God does not promise us a life of ease—even though it seems that some of us are blessed in that way. Everyone faces adversity in life and it's up to each of us to decide how to handle it. We can either rely on our own strength or God's. I know there are people who would rather be "strong" and get through it on their own; but for me, when facing something as life threatening as this, the strength of God is so much more reassuring. It gives you rest and peace. Striving under one's own power is exhausting and I didn't feel I needed to wear myself down any more than necessary—the chemotherapy was doing a good job of that!

The hospital stays were very boring. I tried not to get frustrated and would either read or listen to music on a CD player that Rose had brought me. She supplied a lot of good music to listen to and, at this particular time, I found that to be more enjoyable than reading. It seemed that whenever I would try to read, the aides would come in to make up the bed, my vitals would need to be taken, or some other interruption would occur. It was difficult for me to focus on reading anything other than my Bible. I also think my attention span and retention ability were affected by all the drugs coursing through me! One of the most enjoyable diversions was watching "Survivor." It was a welcome distraction and even now when I hear the theme music I remember those nights in the hospital.

THE POWER OF PRAYER

Many people were praying for me: my family, friends at work and people I didn't even know. Some days it seemed I could actually feel the power of all the prayers being offered on my behalf. Other days I couldn't feel a thing but that didn't stop me from knowing that the prayer power was still there. I truly believe there was a mighty spiritual battle being fought during that time.

One day when Rose was out walking, she thought of Moses standing on the hill when the Israelites were fighting the Amalekites (see Exodus 17: 8-13). In her mind's eye she saw me trying to hold up my arms of faith while Jesus fought against the cancer (as Joshua did against the Amalekites) and decided to ask our good friend who lives in Kentucky to help her hold up my arms. So, as Aaron and Hur helped Moses, they helped me when my faith faltered. She also constantly prayed for legions of angels to surround my bed, the hospital and to be posted outside my hospital room as a hedge of protection. We knew that we were dealing not only with a physical enemy but also a spiritual one.

6

"God is our refuge and strength, an ever-present help in trouble.
Therefore we will not fear."
Psalm 46:1-2

<u>*Journal Entry—Friday, June 16 (at home)*</u>

I had a hard time sleeping last night. I think part of it was getting sick yesterday and losing my meds right after I'd taken them—plus my schedule's all out of whack. I was listening to the birds around 5:00 this morning. They have a little ritual in feeding their babies that I never paid attention to before. As the mother calmed her babies, her lullaby seemed to soothe me also. When we look at the birds and see how God takes care of them, why do we worry and strive so hard?

<u>*Saturday, June 17*</u>

I slept better last night but I'm in some kind of a funk today. I was sick again and that doesn't help. Just getting tired of the chemo, wigs, hospitals, shots and meds, I guess. Went for a short walk—about 15 minutes. I know that's bothering me also. I miss walking and just feeling good. I tried not to stay in a mood too long. I'm also trying not to anticipate my next chemo and hospital stays. Even though I'm about halfway through this ordeal, it seems like it will never end. So, just a day at a time—like the birds. I'll try to focus on just this day. Thank you, Jesus, for watching over me and forgive me for my negative thoughts today.

HALFWAY MARK

The three-week reprieve was a godsend. I was so worn down from the chemotherapy treatments, hair loss trauma and fatigue. My doctor told me I'd start to feel normal again about the third week. I wasn't sure I even remembered what "normal" felt like! Everything was such a blur during this whole time. Days ran together and weeks were melting into months. It had been only about two months since my accident and only one month since my treatments had started. In some ways it felt like only yesterday—in other ways it felt like it had been years.

I tried to keep focused on the fact that I was halfway through the treatment regimen. I knew, however, that the next round would be difficult after having this time off. I just wanted to quit and get back to my life. Being able to be home was great and I knew I'd really have to force myself to go back to the hospital when the time came. I kept thinking about the birds I'd heard that Friday morning. Although I'd been unconsciously aware of them before, their whole existence now seemed to be just for my benefit. I reflected on the soothing song the mother bird sang to her hungry babies and thought of how God sings over us (Zephaniah 3:17). I also remembered what Jesus said about not one sparrow falling without His knowing (Matt. 10:29-31). I reminded myself how much He cares for all His creation and is especially close to those of us who belong to Him. It gave me comfort even in the midst of this dark trial.

Another verse that continued to help me was Psalm 31:14-16: "But I trust in you, O Lord; I say, 'You are my God.' My times are in your hands." I knew in my heart that my life was a clear picture to God even before I was born, but my head and emotions were constantly at war with that truth. Sometimes I felt as though I was my own worst enemy—even worse than the cancer that was trying to destroy me. I knew that if my faith failed—if I gave in to the fear and doubt that plagued me in waves—I could lose it all. I reminded myself of the fact that "Faith is the assurance of things unseen" (Hebrews 11:1). I couldn't see the health I knew God wanted for me, so faith was all I had. I couldn't give in to the fear. I had to trust that even if He took me home, I would stand before Him healthy. Either way, His word would stand true. My part was to trust and believe. Sometimes it was a very hard thing to do.

COMPLAINING

We all have a tendency to complain—it seems to be in our nature. We grumble about traffic, the weather, waiting in line at the grocery store, etc. It's nothing unique but modern society seems to have made it into an art form. Like spoiled children we want everything our own way—and fast! We want it right now—or ten minutes ago. This experience was to be a huge lesson in patience for me. I can grumble and complain with the best of them and I can be just as impatient as the next person. This ordeal seemed to be an excellent opportunity for me to do both—and badly! But for some reason (that can only be explained as the presence of the Holy Spirit) I found that most of the time I wasn't too impatient and wasn't even complaining all that much. Of course, I had my moments. The hospital stays were my greatest tests as I was always ready to leave before I even got into my room! But, for the most part, I was surprised to realize that complaining and impatience just didn't seem appropriate. When I'd see people carrying on in traffic, blowing their horns and waving their arms around in frustration or shifting impatiently from one foot to the other at the checkout counter, I thought about the lessons I was learning.

Complaining is the denial of God's grace. It's denying his omniscience and all-powerful presence in our lives. It can also be an expression of self-pity that, in turn, is a form of idolatry. Our focus is self-centered and on our situations rather than on God and His provision. This is an easy habit to fall into. If we truly believe that God is in control, we commit a serious error when we complain about where we are or what is happening to us. We need to learn 1 Peter 5:7 and Psalm 55:22 and apply them to our daily lives.

I once read that life is 10 percent what happens to us and 90 percent how we respond to it. How we choose to react to circumstances can set the stage for blessing or disaster. Like Paul and Silas when they were in prison, we can sing praises and take what appears to be a bad situation and turn it around into something quite wonderful. Or we can bemoan our lot in life, be miserable and make everyone around us miserable as well.

A THANKFUL HEART

During my illness I found that I usually had to make an effort in reminding myself to be thankful. I tried to remember to be grateful for the little things I <u>could</u> do instead of getting discouraged and depressed over the things I couldn't. During the times I was hospitalized, I tried to be thankful for being able to walk outside—even if it was just around the courtyard with my ever-present walking companion, my IV pole. If it was too hot or raining, I'd go down to the lounge and sit in the recliner chair—I was thankful for that. Sometimes I'd just sit in my hospital room, grateful to be able to look out the window while listening to music.

The Oncology floor had two wings: one faced the courtyard and one faced the parking lot near the main entrance to the hospital. During my seven stays, I had the dubious pleasure of being in several rooms in both wings. When I was in the one facing the courtyard I could watch birds fly back and forth to the birdhouses. When I was in the other wing, I watched people coming in and out of the hospital. Some were laughing, carrying balloons or presents and I'd wonder if they were welcoming a new life. Others would be clutching tissues and dabbing their eyes and I'd wonder if they were saying a final goodbye. I tried to use this time to pray for them and those they were visiting. I even got to know the lawn guy's schedule and enjoyed the wonderful smell of fresh cut grass. I wondered if he knew how lucky he was to be in good health and not in the hospital, and I'd take the opportunity to pray for him too. God always seemed to point out someone to pray for.

7

"Come to me, all you who are weary and burdened, and I will give you rest. Take my yoke upon you and learn from me, for I am gentle and humble in heart, and you will find rest for your souls. For my yoke is easy and my burden is light."
Matthew 10:28-30

Journal Entry—Friday, June 23

I haven't written anything for about a week so this is catch-up time. Karen came over Tuesday night and brought about six videos for me to watch. We had a nice visit. She's going on vacation and I'm trying not to be jealous but sometimes it's hard. On Wednesday (June 21) my sister Mary and I went to a "Look Good, Feel Better" workshop for cancer patients. I think she enjoyed herself and felt like she was helping me some. I was glad to have her with me. It was kind of fun! Yesterday was my birthday and Rose took the day off to spend it with me. I really appreciated that. She tried to make it special and she did, although we didn't know I was going to have a platelet transfusion until late Wednesday and we ended up making three trips to the clinic on my birthday. I praise God that it could be done on an outpatient basis and I didn't have to stay in the hospital. I feel better than I did yesterday so I guess it worked.

I have a CT scan scheduled for July 5 and an appointment with My doctor the following Monday. I'm praying for a good report.

Tuesday, July 11

I'm thanking and praising God for the news yesterday: the tumor is 99% gone and the spinal fluid is still clear! Even though the news is so good, my doctor still wants to continue and finish the protocol, which means three more rounds of treatment with more hospital stays. I just want to get this whole thing over with. At least I get to do this week's treatments at the clinic as an outpatient—it's sure better than the hospital!

Friday, July 14

I'm feeling very weak and tired after a week of chemo. My doctor was right when he said after my three weeks off I'd start to feel like myself again. I did—and now I'm back to being tired all the time and as weak as a kitten. I'm glad I had that time to recuperate a little, though. I was even able to get in a few longer walks. That was nice.

I thank God every day for Rose and all she does for me. I don't think I could get through this by myself. Of course, I know Jesus is always with me and I'm never alone, but it really helps that she's here all the time. Just having someone to help with the little basic things means so much. She's been running errands for me, and taking excellent care of me.

CANCELED PLANS AND NEW ROUTINES

Rose and I had planned a two-week trip to Yosemite National Park in May that had to be cancelled when I received my diagnosis. We speculated on what might have happened if we hadn't found out about the cancer. Could I have collapsed as we were hiking? Rose told me she'd envisioned having to leave me on the trail as she went for help. The scenarios were frightening and, once again, we saw and were grateful for God's hand in this entire situation. Having to cancel our long-planned and much anticipated vacation had been difficult and it was hard not to be jealous of Karen and other friends as they talked about their upcoming trips. I had to constantly speak my heart to Jesus and turn it over to Him. It was a difficult time.

Rose had picked up some information on the *Look Good, Feel Better* workshop for cancer patients that took place at the hospital. She suggested it might be something my sister Mary and I would enjoy. As I noted in my journal, it turned out to be fun as we discussed make-up suggestions, hat and wig ideas. It was informative and also helped to see others going through experiences similar to mine. One woman was brave enough to take her wig off in front of everyone. I could never get to that point. I wore my wig all the time when I went out in public, but at home—and when I was in the hospital—I wore my hats. Many improvements have been made in wigs but I still found it hot and uncomfortable. Sometimes when I was out walking, I just wanted to rip it off—but, of course, I never did.

The opportunity to have even one round of treatment done as an outpatient was a real blessing. It meant a lot of running to and from the clinic every day but I didn't mind. It was much better than having to stay in the hospital. Still, it took its toll and before long I was again feeling run down and tired all the time. Short walks and even going up and down the stairs completely wore me out. I was getting frustrated and depressed. Little did I know it would get a lot worse before it got any better. It's certainly a good thing we can't see into the future. I don't know if I could have gone on had I known what was coming.

SEIZE THE DAY

Carpe Diem—it's become a cliché in society today, but for me it's almost a daily mantra. As I write this in March 2003, it's a windy, late winter day with temperatures near 60 degrees. In the past, I might have complained about the wind—roaring at about 20-25 mph—but not today. I'm thankful that I was able to go for a walk and strong enough to withstand the gusts. I enjoyed feeling the wind whip through my hair braiding it into knots when just 18 months ago I would have been concerned about my wig blowing off. I treasure the soft earth, the grass on the verge of turning green again and the birds celebrating the advent of spring. I seize this day and thank God for granting me another spring to enjoy.

NEW SIGHT

More and more I realize that my spiritual eyesight isn't quite what it should be. This became especially clear to me during my illness. Each morning I would look at myself in the mirror and see the reflection of someone who was sick: thin and pale, sunken cheeks, no hair. Sometimes it would surprise me because there were times that I didn't feel all that bad. It reminded me that often our appearance doesn't accurately reflect how we feel inside. As we get older, each wrinkle we see seems to taunt us with the inevitability of age. No amount of creams can stop the tide of time—and a serious illness often seems to accelerate the process.

I began focusing not on the temporary illness and loss of hair, but on the eternal benefits this experience was providing. I was learning how to lean more fully on Jesus—His love, grace and mercy. I found myself praying more—for other patients, the doctors and nurses. I started telling myself that this wasn't going to last forever, it was just a momentary setback. I found the verses in 2 Corinthians 4:16-18 to be especially appropriate. Even those of us who aren't sick are indeed "outwardly wasting away yet renewed inwardly day by day. So we fix our eyes not on what is seen, but on what is unseen. For what is seen is temporary, but what is unseen is eternal." I may be getting older and may sometimes get sick, but I'm also being spiritually renewed. In essence, I'm becoming younger spiritually—not in my understanding but in strength. As I experience more of life I come to understand, little by little, the things of Heaven and what's really important—what's going to last. In the light of eternity, my troubles down here are minuscule (even though they may not seem so at the time) and will most likely be forgotten when I finally look into Jesus' face.

I used to enjoy camping and the picture Paul presents in the fifth chapter of 2 Corinthians is a wonderful example of things temporal. When you camp, your tent is your temporary home. You put it up and take it down—usually with ease—and when you leave there's little evidence that you've been there at all. That's the way we need to look at our lives here: we're just staying in this campground for a short time. Soon we'll be able to pack up this battered, musty old tent and trade it in for a beautiful house built by Jesus Himself! I long to keep the eyes of my heart constantly fixed on what is eternal.

8

"My heart is in anguish. The terror of death overpowers me. Fear and trembling over-whelm me. I can't stop shaking. Oh, how I wish I had wings like a dove; then I would fly away and rest! I would fly far away to the quiet of the wilderness."
Psalm 55:4-7 (New Living Translation)

Journal Entry—Tuesday, July 18

I'm back in the hospital for the 24-hour methotrexate drip—nasty stuff. The last time I had this it caused a fairly bad outbreak of mouth and throat sores. I hope that doesn't happen again. It's hard enough to eat anything with the food tasting the way it does—but the sores make it so much worse.

Wednesday, July 19

Didn't sleep worth a darn last night. Maybe tonight will be better, but I'm not so sure since I have to take those bicarbonate pills every 3 hours for 48 hours straight. I hope I can at least go back to sleep and that I don't get sick on this stuff. The meals today have been pitiful. I called Rose and asked her to bring me some soup. I'm sure she will. This has been a long day so far and it's only 2:50 p.m. The blessing is that Jean is my nurse through Friday, at which time I hope I can go home.

This morning my doctor said I have no white blood cells! That bothered me but didn't seem to bother him too much. I guess it's to be expected with all this chemo I'm getting. Everyone who comes in has to wash their hands and if I go out of my room I have to wear a facemask. I feel ridiculous wandering the halls like that but I have to get up and move around and can't risk picking up any airborne germs. We got started a little later than usual because the night nurse needed to check with my doctor about my treatments. He's following his protocol all the way.

Monday, July 24 (entries now begin from Rose's journal)

Where is the time and summer going? Joan is home after an upsetting Thursday and an even worse Friday in the hospital. She wasn't released until Saturday because of the toxicity levels. Her doctor explained that the big dose of methotrexate she's getting is to make sure it goes through the spinal fluid and brain. She has to be closely monitored because she could go into a coma if her toxicity levels are over "1" (her level on Friday was 2.1!) The delay in getting out was tough to take, but after he explained the reason, we adjusted our attitudes and looked toward Saturday.

However, another problem has appeared: mouth sores—not new (she had them before) but this time they're much worse. Nothing seems to help and now she's taking morphine to help with the pain. Her white blood cells need to come up—and fast please, Jesus—for the sores to start clearing up. She's so miserable and there's not a thing I can do for her to make it any better.

Please, Jesus, protect Joan from all harm and help her feel better quickly. What I read today in Ruth 3:11 gives me hope: "And now, my daughter, don't be afraid. I will do for you all you ask."

Tuesday, July 25

After taking Joan back to the hospital early this morning (1:00 a.m.) and visiting her three times today, I'm ready for a good night's sleep.

The mouth sores are still bad and now her port may be infected. This must be because of the low white blood cell count. I pray to Jesus that the big doses of antibiotics will bring relief to her tomorrow and that her white count comes up so that she can fight off these mouth sores. She can hardly swallow water and was badly dehydrated when admitted this morning. I feel so sorry for her. If I feel this badly, I can't imagine how Jesus' heart is breaking. Please make her well, Lord. In your compassion please touch her with your healing hand and continue to surround her with the protection of your angels. Watch over her tonight, please, Jesus.

Saturday, July 29

It's 2:00 a.m. and I'm so upset right now I'm not sure I'll get any sleep tonight—or should I say this morning? Joan's terrible experience last night won't soon be forgotten. She was doing pretty well earlier in the evening until that horrible choking episode. She was scared and so was I. Where was Jesus? Why did He let that happen? What was the point? I'm sure that's just something else "we may never know." I'm so glad I was there with her when it happened. I stayed until 1:00 to make sure she was OK and calm enough that she might get some sleep. I don't know if I can ask for anything anymore. It's like I told Derl: if a child asks his father for bread, would he give him a stone? (Matthew 7:8-9) I wonder. This was a pretty stony night.

Sunday, July 30

I'm feeling better tonight than when I made my last entry. Joan's doing much better. She was getting a transfusion when I left. I hope she gets a good night's sleep tonight. I'm praying that her blood counts continue to improve and that she can come home on Wednesday. She really needs to regain her strength and bounce back a bit before this last round of chemo. I thank Jesus again for getting her through this latest ordeal. Even though there's more I wish He would do (like somehow fix this IV problem) I'm grateful for what He's done—seen and unseen. I pray for a good week.

DOWN FOR THE COUNT

This was the beginning of a truly frightening time. My resistance was down and my whole body was reacting to the effects of the toxic drugs I was receiving. Intended to kill the cancer, I wasn't sure they weren't also going to kill me in the process.

The chemo was doing quite a job on my blood levels. I was really scared when I had no white blood cells. I knew this was an extremely dangerous position to be in—any little germ could invade my body and send me into a crisis. Whenever my white count was low I couldn't have any fresh flowers in my hospital room or at home and couldn't eat any fresh vegetables or fruit. As I mentioned in my journal, everyone had to wash their hands before coming into my room and when I ventured out for a walk—even in the halls—I had to wear a mask over my nose and mouth. Trying to keep our humor intact, Rose nicknamed me "the Frito Bandito."

This fifth round of treatments was, I think, the worst. I grudgingly went in Monday evening, July 17, and wanted so badly to go home on Thursday. It was unrealistic but I couldn't help it. I was so discouraged, tired and sick of being sick. I'm afraid I gave the nurses a bit of a hard time. I knew I was being bratty but I didn't care—I just wanted to go home! However, once I realized the ramifications of being released too soon I forced myself to calm down. It was hard but Rose tried her best to cheer me up and we both looked forward to Saturday.

The mouth sores that result from the methotrexate treatments are terrible. The first time I went through it was bad enough but this time, with my resistance and strength worn down, I developed a particularly nasty case of mouth and throat ulcers—stomatitis. No amount of saline rinsing or other treatments helped. I couldn't eat and even liquids were difficult to swallow. I was losing weight and becoming seriously dehydrated. I felt so bad and just wanted to stay at home but in my heart I knew that I needed fluids—and I knew the only way I could keep hydrated was intravenously. I finally gave in and ended up back in the hospital on July 25 after being out for only three days. But, again, God was going before me and there was a bed available at 1:00 a.m. They immediately started me on liquids and antibiotics. The port that had been put in for my treatments was also infected so they weren't able to use it at all. That meant more poking with needles for the IVs. My veins have never been that good and the chemotherapy was damaging them even more, so it was difficult for the technicians and nurses to find a vein to use. Some of the attempts were extremely painful and, as a result, I had bruises all over my arms.

I was finally starting to feel better on Thursday and mentioned it to Rose when she came up to see me. Not long after that I was given some liquid medicine that sent me into a violent coughing spell. My throat was on fire and I couldn't catch my breath. I ended up on oxygen because my blood oxygen level fell. It took me over two hours to recover. That episode caused my throat to become badly inflamed again and lengthened my stay in the hospital.

WHEN THERE'S NO ANSWER

God wants us to learn to trust Him and sometimes His answer to our pleas isn't what we want to hear. I believe He could have miraculously cured me—or at least kept me from going through everything I did. The complications that came from the treatments could have been avoided had He seen fit to allow it. For some reason He didn't and I had to endure His will. I often thought of Jesus in the garden the night before His death, pleading with His Father for the cup to pass—but it was not to be and He had to listen to the silence as we sometimes do. These are the times we must, in faith, accept His answer and not misunderstand or misinterpret His intention. It is through the periods of darkness—not by some miraculous deliverance—that we learn to trust Him and His word. These times of testing actually help us to grow (more than the times of blessing) and, as we do, we learn that sometimes His best answer to our prayers and pleadings is a soft, loving "No." His ways are always better and if He is sometimes silent, we can be sure He has something better in mind for us. It might not become apparent right away (it certainly didn't to me) but eventually we will look back and see His graciousness and our resulting growth in Him.

9

"My God, my God, why have you forsaken me? Why are you so far from saving me, so far from the words of my groaning? O my God, I cry out by day, but you do not answer, by night and am not silent."
Psalm 22:1-2

Friday, August 4 *(entries continue from Rose's journal)*

Joan's illness is weighing both of us down. I'm so worried about her. I know it's a sin to worry but I pray and pray and she just seems to get worse. I'm afraid to pray anymore. I don't even know what to pray for. I'm afraid to get my hopes up—afraid of what might happen. I know that fear is a powerful tool of Satan and I'm not supposed to give in to it. I know that I'll feel fear but I can't allow it to control me. I have to keep trusting God and believing in Him—that He's in control and knows what He's doing. I pray I can do that.

Tuesday, August 8

I cry out in desperation to my Lord on behalf of my sister in Christ—and his child—Joan. My cries for compassion and mercy are continuous before His throne. I ask for an end to the trials and tests (and punishment?) and an outpouring of His mercy and compassion. I ask for small miracles from a big God. Is that my mistake? I know He hears—I pray His answer is "Yes."

It's 11:35 p.m. and I just got home from the hospital. There were small miracles for Joan tonight. Please, Jesus, have this be the victory over this enemy—no more procedures, no more vomiting. Give her the ability to tolerate a progressive diet. Heal her, please, of this latest setback. Have the blockage problem be solved and no more bile back ups. The promise of Ruth 3:11 seems dim—yet I cling to it.

Wednesday, August 9

Another day and no more miracles—little or big. My flesh and every ounce of my spirit longs to lash out in bitterness and rage. But all I can muster is a feeble display of frustration and anger—and then I confess my sin and again try to turn this whole situation over to Jesus. Our talk with Pam (the nursing technician) tonight helped somewhat. I should have stayed with Joan tonight at the hospital. I feel bad that I didn't. I will tomorrow night—she may need me more then. Lord Jesus, please show us some mercy and compassion!

Friday, August 11

Thank you, Jesus! After a shaky start—Joan's IG tube came out as she was getting washed up—her surgery was moved up from 6:30 p.m. to 4:00 with Joan finally going in around 5:00 p.m. It was a long day. The surgery went fine and the obstruction was apparently just scar tissue. I pray her recovery is quick and complete. I was such an emotional wreck as I walked with her to pre-op. I'm sure people thought I was nuts but I couldn't control it. I'm afraid I wasn't much moral or spiritual support for her—at least not until I finally got myself pulled together (thank you, Holy Spirit.) Spending last night at the hospital and only getting a couple of hours of sleep probably didn't help, but still. Whatever is wrong with me? I thank God that He watched over Joan and guided the surgeon's hand.

THE DARKEST HOUR

Things seemed to go from bad to worse. I finally got out of the hospital (again!) on Thursday, August 3 ready to go home but still not feeling that good. The mouth sores were responding to the antibiotics and I had been receiving fluids and nourishment intravenously. I was even able to get down some broth and soft food so I knew I was improving.

I was only home for about a day, however, when I started vomiting green bile. At first, I thought it was a reaction to the morphine they had given me to relieve the pain of the mouth and throat sores. It continued through the day on Friday and all through the night. By Saturday morning, August 5, I could barely get from the couch to the bathroom—which was not more than 10-15 feet away. Rose was scared and called my sister to help get me back to the hospital. When Mary got there, she and Rose decided they weren't able to get me down the stairs and I ended up being taken in by ambulance.

Because of the vomiting I was again becoming badly dehydrated and the attendants couldn't get a blood pressure reading on me when I was sitting up. Once more, a bed was miraculously available and I was admitted immediately. (This was unusual since the Oncology floor of the hospital is always full—but every time I needed a bed, God seemed to have gone before me and had one waiting.)

X-rays and CT scans were run the next day and it was discovered that I had some sort of intestinal blockage. The doctors couldn't be sure whether or not it was a new tumor or scar tissue from the gall bladder surgery I'd had 30 years ago. The thought of a possible new tumor had me really scared. In addition, my doctor was urging me to have a NG tube inserted in order to drain the bile. I hated the thought of it and fought it for as long as I could. My nurses also encouraged me to have the procedure done. I finally relented on Wednesday, August 9. Rose walked the grounds of the hospital praying fervently that it would go well. This period of time was extremely hard on her emotionally and, while I was concerned that she was wearing herself down, I was very grateful for her constant presence and support.

Thursday was an especially difficult day. There were more x-rays and consultations with doctors. The thought that the cancer might have shown up again and in a different place had both Rose and me very concerned. She decided to spend the night at the hospital and I was glad for her company. At 10:00 that night my oncologist was kind enough to call the nurses and ask them to let me know that the blockage did not appear to be a new tumor. About an hour later, another doctor came in to tell me that they were scheduling me for exploratory surgery the next day. At this point, Rose and I knew that neither one of us would get much sleep that night. It was a fitful night, broken only by the scheduled vitals checks and medications distributed by the nurses. When Friday morning finally dawned it felt as though a week had passed and we both looked pretty ragged. I faced a long day and I was still scared about the surgery and what it might reveal.

FACING FEAR

The situation seemed to be spinning out of control—spiraling downward. Things would go along fairly smoothly and then a setback would kick out all the props I'd been leaning on—all but one: Jesus. Fear, which was a constant presence and almost overwhelming by now, would send me running to Him and the comfort of His arms. I knew that it was normal to experience the anxiety of what was happening to me but I also knew that to give in to worry and fear was sin. I couldn't let it control me. This, I think, was one of the hardest lessons to learn. Nothing helped so much as the prayers of my friends and the verses I had memorized.

During this time I was becoming especially conscious of the Holy Spirit's role in my life. We often fall into a routine of praying to Jesus or to our Heavenly Father but rarely do we think about the miraculous presence of the Holy Spirit in our hearts. I became acutely aware of the reality of Romans 8:26,27—"In the same way, the Spirit helps us in our weakness. We do not know what we ought to pray for, *but the Spirit himself intercedes for us with groans that words cannot express*. And He who searches our hearts knows the mind of the Spirit, because the Spirit intercedes for the saints *in accordance with God's will*" (emphasis added). At this point, neither Rose nor I knew what to pray for. It seemed as though nothing was happening the way we thought it should. But we found comfort in the knowledge that the Holy Spirit was interceding for us since we were literally at a loss for words.

I was relieved and my prayers were answered when the doctors found only scar tissue, just as they had suspected. However, the following week was one of the worst for me. I had to stay up on the surgery floor where I didn't know any of the nurses and they didn't know me. I desperately missed being down with my "family" in Oncology. There were many "code blue" calls while I was there (one for the room right next to mine) and fear was almost a tangible presence. I was completely at the end of myself. Oddly enough I think that I was more scared during this time than at any other. I had nightmares that the cancer was back and would wake up shaking and in a cold sweat. The combination of the pain from the surgery and the medication given to relieve it had me doubting whether I'd ever get out of there alive. But I finally did, and the happiness I had felt when I was released from previous hospital stays paled significantly when compared to when I got home this time.

10

"You hem me in—behind and before; you have laid your hand upon me. Where can I go from your Spirit? If I make my bed in the depths, you are there. Even there, your hand will guide me, your right hand will hold me fast."
Psalm 139: 5, 7-10

Tuesday, August 22 (entries continue from Rose's journal)

Well, we've passed some significant milestones in the past few days. Successful surgery, a few days of post-surgery stress, then Joan's discharge. We had a shaky first night home that resulted in me getting on my face (literally) before God and pleading for her healing. I claimed every verse in the Bible that referred to heal, healed, healing, etc. She's slowly but steadily getting stronger and passed the "test" of being home for five full days. I thank God for all He's done. I look forward to it continuing and just getting better and better. Even though Joan's experiencing some fairly serious anxiety attacks and fear about the future, Jesus is helping me to encourage her to believe and trust—believe that He can take care of us and trust that He'll do it. Just trust Him. We truly must have the faith of a child.

Saturday, September 2

Labor Day weekend—I can hardly believe it! I'm switching between two football games and Joan's on the balcony giving herself a manicure. It's good to have her home. She's concerned about the week's delay before her last treatment. We're praying and believing God for the complete healing we've claimed. He's true to His word and we can trust Him. I, for one, can't let <u>anyone</u> (not even Joan) influence me on this. I am determined to stand firm and continue to hold up her arms of faith in the strength the Holy Spirit gives me.

A SHORT RECUPERATION

This was a relatively calm period of time except for the first couple of weeks after the surgery. I found myself dealing with a lot of fear and anxiety and I seemed to worry about every little thing—my insurance, my job and the long-term ramifications of this whole experience. I don't know if it was the culmination of everything that had happened to me, the effects of all the drugs I'd been on, or something else. Whatever the cause, I probably had more difficulty thinking clearly and keeping things in perspective at this time than at any other during the entire ordeal.

The trauma of the past month had taken its toll. Rose and I were both exhausted and used the weeks between my surgery and my last scheduled treatment to rest and recuperate. (She had left her job for three months to take on the full-time responsibility of my care. It turned out to be a wise decision. She was invaluable to me during my recovery from the unexpected surgery and now she was able to regroup and get some much-needed rest.) Neither one of us had much energy so our activities were limited to just the basics. I worked on building my strength after the surgery by taking short walks. I was enjoying the late summer weather immensely and trying not to think of the final treatment that still loomed before me. Actually, I was hoping that it might be canceled, and I even tried to talk my doctor into doing so—but no such luck! He wasn't about to leave this unfinished and was intent on completing his protocol. It was only postponed an extra week to give me a little more time to heal. I was concerned about the effects of the chemotherapy on my incision, since every part of the body is affected by the treatments. I tried not to worry and reminded myself that God had gotten me this far. I had to trust Him to take me all the way through.

LEARNING FROM TULIPS

Although I continued to read daily from my Bible and thanked God each day for His care, the intensity level dropped considerably during this time. My reliance on Jesus during the past 4-1/2 months had been almost frantic and the relative calm that I now felt almost seemed wrong. I realized, however, that although the emotional aspect had changed, the depth hadn't.

Sometimes when we are in the midst of a crisis, every other part of our life becomes almost insignificant. We can't be bothered with things that once seemed so important—all else pales next to the enormity of what's facing us. Our whole perspective changes when faced with matters of life and death. Things we once took for granted or deemed trivial, like the sound of birds singing or the shapes of the clouds, are now seen through appreciative eyes. When things calm somewhat, we may not talk to God as desperately as before but, as we enjoy and appreciate the everyday gifts He gives, our hearts send out a song of praise to the one who holds everything together. We often allow our busy lives to rob us of the joy of experiencing life; but when faced with the possibility of dying, life itself becomes much more real.

I once read that if you make a tiny slit in the stem of a tulip right beneath the flower, it won't droop so quickly when put into water. Apparently, the flower directs its energy toward healing the wound instead of opening more fully. Therefore, the flower stays upright and fresh looking longer. I found this fascinating. The injury actually causes the flower to flourish! Its beauty—and even its life—is prolonged. I tried to look at my own situation in a similar light. I was certainly wounded and had to decide where my strength and energy were going to go—toward repairing the wound or toward worry and self-pity. Sometimes God "wounds" us in loving discipline. Other times it might be just to make us strong and more like Him. In either case, I often tried to remind myself that Jesus was with me, that He promised never to leave me (John 14:16-18 and Hebrews 13:5-6) and, like Joshua, I need not be afraid nor discouraged. Admittedly, this is easier said than done. But I had the Holy Spirit inside to give me strength when mine failed.

DAY-BY-DAY

I find it interesting that Jesus' first recorded miracle was not a healing, but took place at a party—a time of joy. In this, He demonstrated His concern for the totality of our lives—His interest in the every day details, not just the crises. This shows me that He's interested not only in my needs—which He promises to meet—but also my wants. I sometimes find, though, that when things calm down and the immediate crisis has passed, I assume He's moved on to something bigger, someone else's crisis. Yes, He's able to do that but He also stays with me—when my life again becomes routine—and walks with me through my "dailies."

I've read about the Israelites' wanderings after leaving Egypt and I shake my head in wonder how, after miracle upon miracle, they started complaining when they returned to daily living. But then I remember that I'm guilty of much the same thing. Sometimes the "daily-ness" of my everyday life hinders my ability to see God in everything—sometimes I have to look a bit harder. But, if I can learn to remember that He's always with me, every minute of my life can be wonderful—not just the exciting times when He's moving mountains for me.

11

"I waited patiently for the Lord; He turned to me and heard my cry. He lifted me out of the slimy pit, out of the mud and mire; He set my feet on a rock and gave me a firm place to stand. He put a new song in my mouth, a hymn of praise to our God."
Psalm 40:1-3

Friday, September 15 *(this entry is from Joan's journal)*

Today is the end of a pretty uneventful week—the last of my chemo treatments—and I hope it stays that way. We got started at least an hour later than usual. Patient endurance seems to be my lesson through this. I've been praying about the spinal tomorrow and hope everything goes smoothly. Should be the last one!

My hair is starting to come back—just "peach fuzz" right now but it's nice to see. I hope this last treatment doesn't make it come out again.

I thank God every day for my body's reaction to this whole chemo regimen. Aside from the mouth sores it's gone pretty well. Rose overheard some women talking about how sick they were getting from drugs and doses that weren't half as strong as mine. All in all, I think I've only gotten sick about 5 times from the chemo itself. I know that it's only by God's grace I've done that well. Thank you, Jesus!

Tuesday, October 3 *(remaining entries are from Rose's journal)*

Things continue to move along, although Joan and I have each experienced our own little "funk"—Joan's being due to some hair loss (darn!) resulting from the final chemo treatment and mine being uncertainty about going back to my job and dealing with a nagging eye problem. I'm hoping the eye thing is minor. However, since Joan's diagnosis every pain and deviance from normal is suspect. It's hard not to worry so much—it does no good and, being the opposite of trust and faith, is actually sin. This little valley seems to be the result of the end of a manic and frantic five months. We need to enjoy this time rather than worrying about what may be coming.

Tuesday, October 17

More than two months since Joan's surgery and six months since the accident that started this nightmarish roller coaster ride. We get her CT scan results this Friday and are hoping expectantly for a good report.

Friday, October 20

Thank you, Jesus and Halleluiah! Joan's CT scan shows that the tumor is completely gone. We're both so happy! Now my prayers are for Joan's continued recuperation.

THE FINISH LINE

Going in for my last round of treatment was hard. I'd been out of the hospital for over a month and was starting to feel pretty decent. I was glad, though, that it was only one more treatment. Rose and I continuously talked of seeing God's hand throughout this entire ordeal. He intervened right from the start and never left me—even though, at times, I felt He was far away. In my heart I knew that He was with me through every procedure, that He cried with me when I was so scared I didn't know what to do, and He had gathered all my tears (Psalm 58:8).

As noted in my journal entry, I was pleasantly surprised one morning when I noticed the "peach fuzz" on my head. Could it be that my hair was actually starting to come back? But what would happen when I had my last treatment? I tried not to think too much about the future and just enjoy what was happening now. My eyebrows and eyelashes were also coming back. I was starting to look like myself again. But, unfortunately, soon after the last treatment, what little hair I had started coming out. It had been about six weeks since I'd had any chemotherapy drugs in my system and now it seemed my body was in a state of shock. I was hoping that this "last little dose" wouldn't cause any fallout but, once again, I underestimated the power of the drugs I was getting. It was pretty much back to square one! I was discouraged and wondered if I'd ever have a full head of hair. It took another 6-8 weeks before it started to grow again and there seemed to be more gray hair than I remembered. (I imagine the stress of the past few months had something to do with that!) The growth process was slow and it wasn't until many months later that I felt comfortable going out in public without my wig.

The next few weeks were spent recuperating and waiting for my next CT scan. I prayerfully anticipated a good report and was rewarded with a happy smile from my doctor. Rose and I rejoiced and turned our focus on getting back to a normal life, although I don't think any part of me will ever be "normal" again.

After my last treatment, my appetite also slowly started returning. At first, the only thing that really appealed to me was a milk shake Rose would prepare using Instant Breakfast (so I'd get some nutrients), ice cream, a banana, milk and crushed ice. My blender was a pretty old one and couldn't handle ice cubes, so Rose ended up putting them in a washcloth and pounding them with a hammer. For the most part it worked pretty well—except once when she lost her concentration and ended up smashing her thumb! We often thought we should have filmed these incidents—they would have been pretty funny to watch in years to come.

IN THE PASTURE

Psalm 23 is probably one of the most well known pieces of writing in the world. I've read and recited it countless times, but have only recently come to a better understanding of it. The comparison of us to sheep with Jesus as the Good Shepherd is not just by chance. There is a wonderful picture here if we understand the characteristics of sheep and the character and role of the shepherd.

Sheep are fairly dumb animals that tend to wander off easily often thinking only of their immediate hunger. The shepherd must actually lead them to the grazing areas that, in Israel, are often quite sparse. There aren't meadows of ankle-high grass where they can graze for days on end. Instead, the "green pastures" are actually mere clumps of grass scattered in a rocky landscape. He guides them along the path providing just enough grazing for the day and doesn't take them anywhere he hasn't gone before. When it begins to get dark, instead of leading them he walks *among* them—talking to them and guiding them to the pen where he himself becomes the "gate," keeping them safe inside and protecting them from predators.

What a wonderful picture this is of our walk with Jesus. I've learned that He does, indeed, lead me beside the quiet waters and guide me along His paths. He's been everywhere I'm going and provides for me every day. He comforts me with his staff and is with me in the shadowy valleys. I don't need to worry about tomorrow—He's already been there.

SAND AND SEED

I often read the "Footprints in the Sand" plaque that hangs on the wall in my bathroom. It's another well-known piece of writing yet, again, it now takes on a new meaning for me. I feel much like the writer who looks back on his life and at times sees only one set of footprints. Jesus carried me through much of this experience. Even though I sometimes felt as if He had deserted me, He was, in fact, carrying me—shouldering the load of my sickness, my small faith and my trembling heart.

Jesus told His disciples that if they had even the tiniest bit of faith they could move mountains. He compared the necessary size of our faith to a mustard seed—one of the smallest seeds known. I've realized it's the *object* of our faith—not the size—that is most important. Our faith and trust must be in the

One who cares for us so much that He was willing to set aside eternal fellowship with His Father and take on a weak, human body, walk in this sin-sick world for 33 years and die for us. He's "been there, done that." He's gone before us and is able to carry us through.

12

"Fear not, for I have redeemed you; I have summoned you by name; you are mine.
When you pass through the waters, I will be with you... When you walk through the
fire, you will not be burned; the flames will not set you ablaze."
Isaiah 43:2

I returned to work in November on a part-time basis and slowly worked my way up to my current 30-hour per week schedule. I still have back pain due to the non-functioning kidney and some arthritis in my spine. My left kidney continues working at only about 10 percent of its capacity and will probably never function normally again.

At times, those six months in 2000 seem like a dream: hazy, clouded with pain and medications, almost surreal. Other times, especially when my back pain is particularly acute, it's all too real. I sometimes ask myself if this disease may actually have been a gift. What did I learn through this experience?

Primarily, I think it made me more sensitive to other people. So often we tend to put places like hospitals, nursing homes and rehabilitation centers out of our minds because they remind us of how fragile life really is and they make us uncomfortable by showing us how vulnerable we are. Of course, it's certainly not healthy to think about these things constantly, but neither should we put them out of our thoughts altogether. We need an even-balanced awareness of the circumstances and needs of others. Often the sick, poor or handicapped are thought of as being less fortunate. But I wonder now if that's really true. Many times those with hardships have a measure of faith, peace and contentment that healthy, comfortable people will never experience.

Sometimes hardships are discipline from God (Hebrews 12: 4-8). But they can also be the testing of our faith—to help us grow into what God knows we can be. Left to our own devices, most of us would choose an easy path to spiritual maturity. But, unless we're firmly rooted in our faith, we'll topple like a tree in shallow soil at the first strong wind of adversity. I know that I've grown through this experience.

GOLD, GRAIN AND A LITTLE CLAY

I am reminded of something I heard about the process of refining gold. It's a story of a man and woman who went to a small shop to buy some gold jewelry. Finding no one in the front of the shop, they went into the back room. There they found the owner intently watching a pot simmering on a fire. He told them he was in the process of refining some gold and couldn't leave it unattended. As he closely monitored the fire, constantly keeping his eye on the refining process, he explained that if the fire got too hot the gold would be destroyed and if it got too cool the gold would harden with all the impurities still in it. They asked him when he knew the refining was complete and he replied, "When I can see my image in it."

I found that to be a wonderful picture of God as the ultimate refiner—constantly watching us through the entire life process, waiting until He finally sees His image in us. We need to remember that whatever trial or hardship we go through, God never takes His eye off us. Whether or not we feel His presence, He never leaves us. He sits with us, watching closely, crying with us and holding us close. "See, I have refined you, though not as silver; I have tested you in the furnace of affliction" (Isaiah 48:10).

And, as Shadrach, Meschach and Abednego were not alone in the fiery furnace, neither are we when we find ourselves in the flames of affliction. God was with them—He will be with us. And when we come out, we will be like them: "the fire had not harmed their bodies, nor was a hair of their heads singed; their robes were not scorched, and there was no smell of fire on them." (Daniel 3:27) Our physical body may be a bit damaged, but our spirit will not be harmed—only strengthened, purified and made more like Jesus.

Like grain, we are sometimes threshed, bruised and crushed in the refining process. But the method is different for each variety of grain. "Caraway is not threshed with a sledge, neither is a cart wheel rolled over cummin; caraway is beaten out with a rod and cummin with a stick. Grain must be ground to make bread; so one does not go on threshing it forever. Though he drives the wheels of his threshing cart over it, his horses do not grind it. All this also comes from the Lord Almighty" (Isaiah 28:27-28). Grain takes a lot of pounding until it becomes fine white powder, ready to be used—but it's not crushed forever. And, as clay on a potter's wheel, we must be still and unresisting, submitting to His every touch. Only then will He be able to fashion us into the beautiful likeness of His Son.

VIEW FROM THE HEIGHTS

In the wonderful allegory *Hinds' Feet in High Places* by Hannah Hurnard, the central character, Much-Afraid, goes on a journey to the High Places with The Shepherd. He sends two companions with her. She's horrified to discover their names are Sorrow and Suffering. At first she refuses their silently offered assistance, but soon realizes their value and they become trusted friends. Together they face many challenges and she learns valuable lessons about fear, pride and loneliness. When they finally reach their destination all three receive new names: Much-Afraid is transformed into Grace and Glory and her companions become Joy and Peace.

I look at my experience with cancer as one of many challenges I am facing on my own journey to the High Places. I can certainly identify with Much-Afraid and I've known Sorrow and Suffering as my traveling companions. I dealt with the "Fearing Invasion" and wandered in the "Forests of Danger and Tribulation." But through it all, as with the character in the book, the Shepherd is always with me—even if I don't see Him—and comes striding joyfully out of the gloom when I call. "The Sovereign Lord is my strength; he makes my feet like the feet of a deer, he enables me to go on the heights" (Habakkuk 3:19).

Even though I've read the book several times and am quite familiar with the story, a unique lesson is learned upon each reading. Sometimes we find ourselves in a place we know we've been before and yet there's something new to be learned—a higher level to reach in our walk with God. With each trial He brings us through He also brings us to a new degree of intimacy with Him and His ways. We can certainly never fully understand the mind or heart of God, but just knowing that He holds our hand and loves us should be enough for us to completely trust what He is doing. He loves us with a reckless, raging fury—so much so that He gave up His only Son for our sake. We broke the covenant and yet He paid the price. Can we put our lives into the hands of a God who did that?

GOD'S FINGERPRINTS

Rose and I saw God's involvement throughout this entire experience—from the accident that found the tumor the doctors were missing, through His protection of me during the chemotherapy treatments and blood transfusions. Even the stomatitis was part of His plan. We firmly believe that had I not developed those bad mouth and throat sores, the intestinal blockage may very well have been discovered during my final treatment. With my blood levels dangerously low and my immune system ravaged by the cancer and the chemotherapy drugs, surgery would have been extremely risky. We are sure that the large doses of antibiotics given to fight off the stomatitis also prevented me from getting a post-surgery infection. Neither of us have any doubt that God was in complete control of the entire situation.

I won't soon forget what I've been through, although at times I find myself falling back into the routine of rushing, worrying and getting upset over little things. I then stop and ask myself, "How serious is this, really? Remembering those months in 2000 helps me keep things in the proper perspective. I pray that my relationship with Jesus will continue to be foremost in my life and that I will continue to value the simple gifts that life brings me every day. If you are going through a hard time right now, please know this: God loves you and He will get you through it. If His eye is on the sparrow, how much more will it be on us, His beloved children? Trust Him.

EPILOGUE

"I will present my thank offerings to you. For you have delivered me from death and my feet from stumbling, that I may walk before God in the light of life."
Psalm 56:12-13

If the year 2000 was a year of trial and testing, 2001 was a year of blessing. The spring and summer were hectic months but nothing like the previous year. After many years of renting, I decided to become a homeowner and in April I bought a condo. The following month Rose and I were blessed to be able to go on our vacation to Yosemite that we had canceled the year before. I think it was even more special for me than it would have been originally. I was awed by the grandeur of what I saw—knowing that the one who created this spectacular beauty was so intimately involved in my life.

Earlier in the year Rose had entered The Leukemia & Lymphoma Society's Team-In-Training for The Midnight Sun Marathon, naming me as her personal hero and, in June, she treated me to a dream trip to Alaska for my 55th birthday. A far cry from the "celebration" of my birthday the previous year, it was a wonderful trip that I'll never forget. About a week after returning, I moved into my new home.

In September 2002 I passed the two-year milestone for this rare type of cancer and, as of February 2004, continue to be cancer-free.

AFTERWORD

"Praise be to the God and Father of our Lord Jesus Christ, the Father of compassion and the God of all comfort, who comforts us in all our troubles, so that we can comfort those in any trouble with the comfort we ourselves have received from God."
2 Corinthians 1:3-4

This verse is the perfect expression of why I have written this book. I believe that the things we experience in life are not only for our benefit and growth but also to help and give comfort to others. If we share our experiences—both good and bad—and the lessons learned through them, we can truly touch someone's life in a remarkable way.

If you have been diagnosed with cancer or any other serious disease, I pray that, as you have read this, God has touched you with His comforting hand and you realize that you are not alone. If you don't know Jesus Christ as your personal Savior and Lord, I invite you to ask Him into your heart. Talk to Him as you would a friend—confessing your fears and shortcomings—then ask Him to take your life and make you more like Him. Your life may not get better immediately. In fact, you may—and probably will—face some difficult times; but you will have the joy of knowing that He will always be there to walk you through. May God richly bless you.

0-595-31252-7

www.ingramcontent.com/pod-product-compliance
Lightning Source LLC
Chambersburg PA
CBHW021257280526
45784CB00005B/2405